ALOE VERA: THE NATURAL HEALER

THE FIRST EVER "USER FRIENDLY" GUIDE TO ALOE VERA.

D0533628

Written & compiled by Paul Hornsey-Pennell,
with contributions from Dr. Peter Atherton.

ALOE VERA: THE NATURAL HEALER

The First Ever "User Friendly" Guide to Aloe Vera

by

Paul Hornsey-Pennell

Published in the U.K. by
The Wordsmith Publishing Company,
46a West Street, Farnham,
Surrey GU9 7DU

First published in 1994

Reprinted 1995 (twice)

Cover photograph courtesy of Forever Living Products (U.K.) Ltd.

ISBN 0 9524645 0 0

Printed in Great Britain by Whitstable Litho Printers,
Whitstable, Kent.

ACKNOWLEDGEMENTS

I would like to thank Dr. Peter Atherton for his knowledge, interest and guidance.

Dr. Gregg Henderson, whose professional account of his many years of experience using Aloe Vera in his practice, provided me with so much information.

Azina Heart, a precious friend whose support through the writing of this book has been invaluable.

Fiona, my wife, for looking after the children all the time while I was writing this book and, in particular, for persuading me to try Aloe Vera.

AUTHOR'S NOTE

The Natural Healer contains accounts of individual experiences and the consequential results of having used Aloe Vera. The reason for writing about them is because of the seemingly inexplicable way(s) in which this plant has helped so many people with so many varying conditions and ailments.

It must be noted, however, that no suggestion is being made that anyone with a medical problem should give up treatment that they may be having, or medication that they may be taking, nor is the information in this book meant to be prescriptive. This book is about observations and opinions, nothing more. It is not intended to be a substitute/replacement for medical advice. If anyone reading this has a medical condition or problem, then consult your doctor.

Caution for diabetics: There is a possibility that the drinking of Aloe Vera juice may increase the amount of insulin that you naturally produce. It is essential that you consult your doctor. *Some diabetics have stated that, since taking Aloe Vera, their insulin requirement has reduced considerably.*

CONTENTS

INTRODUCTION

It wasn't until I actually sat down to write this book that I realised what a challenge and a problem the subject matter, a spiky, green coloured plant called Aloe Vera had presented me with. The challenge was to write about a plant that has the longest known medical association with mankind and how, after 4,000 years, it not only seems to alleviate an A-Z list of medical conditions that the modern drugs of today have scarce impact on but, in addition has refused to yield the secret as to how it does this. Ironically, it is because of the quite extraordinary versatility of the plant, together with the fact that it cannot be fully explained that presents the problem, which is (in)credibility.

As you progress through this book you will read about the properties that are contained in the leaves of this plant, along with a list of ailments and conditions with which it has had repeated success, all backed up by testimonials. You will read words like "remarkable", "extraordinary", "amazing" and "incredible" many times and there may well be moments when I may seem to enthuse to the point of delusion but this is only a combination of passion, lack of self control and a limited vocabulary!

So the way that I see it is that this may well appear too good to be true for some and it is to those people that I would ask, particularly if you are suffering in any way, please read this book with an open mind and when you have done this, then ask yourself what you may be doubting. If you require hard rigid facts that conclusively and scientifically prove how this plant can have such results, then you will not find them in here. There are other books which contain analyses in them but none that will give you a definitive answer as to how Aloe Vera actually does what it does for the simple reason that no-one has been able to come up with one. What this book gives you is evidence and the choice as to whether to accept it or not, which is at the exact place where I found myself eleven months ago.

This is very much a "beginners guide to . . ." book. Any areas that were remotely technical I have attempted to write in as simplistic a way as I can. The reason for this is straight forward. When I started researching into Aloe Vera there were two aspects that weren't right for me. The first was that there was little information around concerning how to take Aloe Vera and in what quantity. Then there was the issue of wanting to know what was in it. I knew that Aloe Vera contained minerals, vitamins, amino acids, enzymes etc. all of which were familiar terms to me but I actually felt a little foolish about not knowing what these things are or do. As I assumed that "everyone knows what these things are", it was a strange comfort to find the truth is that everyone doesn't know what these things are and many people, like me have also felt foolish asking. The consequence of this is that I have attempted to explain not only what is in Aloe Vera but what things like, for instance, proteins do and why we need them. We all know the word protein and that we need to look out for these things in our diet but how many of us know why?

In addition, my writing style is, at times, light hearted. This is not because I don't take this matter seriously. I do. However I am someone who was extremely cynical about what I had been told this plant might do for me, until, that is the day that I needed it. Any light humour, therefore, comes from not only having the quality of my life greatly improved as a *direct* result of using Aloe Vera (see the next chapter) but from a degree of embarrassment as to my initial cynicism!

Having "come clean" as to my medical ignorance, you may be wondering what are my credentials for writing this book? In terms of medical qualifications, I have none and I consider this as my biggest credential of all because it means that I don't have a medical opinion to give. What I do have is personal experience of using Aloe Vera on myself and of witnessing the effect that it has had on family, friends, pets and total strangers. During my research for this book, I came across accounts, both first and second hand, of cases where the individuals concerned had suffered so terribly and for such a long time, having been given up on by "conventional" medicine. They then heard of Aloe Vera and, upon trying it, experienced a relief that they would never have believed possible. I should also add that I am not saying that this has been in every case.

Another "credential" is my cynicism. Obviously my attitude to Aloe Vera has changed but when I was introduced to it by my wife, I was dreadfully scornful. Was I really expected to believe that this Aloe Vera "stuff" was capable of alleviating a list of conditions that, literally, went from A to Z? If this was such a remarkable plant, then how come I'd never heard of it before? etc.

I have what I regard as a healthy suspicion of "orthodox" medicine. This does not mean that I am against it. If I have an immovable headache you will not find me waiting for nature to take its course, you will find me reaching for the painkillers! However, I believe strongly in the body's ability to look after itself and that the best way to heal is to provide it with what it requires not only to induce its own exceptional healing resources but to prevent illness and disease happening in the first instance. "Western" medicine, although awesome in its ability to analyse, seems to me at times to be clumsy, if not brutal, in its implementation, often with a price to pay in the form of a side effect, reflecting an attitude of controlling, rather than complementing what is naturally present.

Finally, my reasons for writing this book are that, firstly, I have no doubt that Aloe Vera possesses properties that hundreds of thousands of people, probably millions, would benefit from. Secondly, I believe that there is a need for more basic information on the more practical aspects of Aloe Vera. Thirdly, I believe that the integration of more natural health care and conventional health care would lead to a healthier health care. Fourth, this book needed writing.

What this book *is not* about is persuasion. It is not about making wild, unsubstantiated claims that Aloe Vera will cure all ills. It is simply about Aloe Vera and people, as it has been for thousands of years. Make of it what you will.

I do hope that you enjoy this book. I would ask that, even if you feel so inclined, please don't simply dismiss it. Why is it that the human condition, in its thirst for answers, so often becomes blind to reality?

Above all else, what I hope for is relief for those who are suffering.

CHAPTER ONE
ME, MY FAMILY &
ALOE VERA

In December 1993, I, along with thousands of others in the U.K., was suffering from "Beijing flu", with the unpleasant additions of sinusitis, a highly inflamed and very painful ear infection and a throat that felt as though it had been skinned on the inside. I was into day four and, having suffered the indignity of an injection in my right buttock to relieve the migraine caused by the pressure of the sinusitis, I looked and felt wretched.

It was at this moment that Fiona, my wife, came into the room with a little bottle in her hand. It was obvious from the moaning and snuffling that was coming out from under the duvet that I was in my "I would greatly appreciate everyone staying at least a hundred and twenty five miles away from me and, on your way out, don't forget to cancel Christmas!" mood! Fiona, by now quite used to the "Don't you know that I'm dying?" routine, put the bottle by me saying that as it would appear that the injection had had no effect then what about trying some Aloe Vera? "Aloe what?" I snuffled, "Aloe Vera" replied Fiona, "apparently, if you were to squeeze some up your nose and down your ear, it might well ease the pain." Patronisingly, I scoffed at the idea, asking if she really thought that this Aloe "stuff" had any chance of success where the doctor's drugs had failed? With the answer, "What have you got to lose?" Fiona left the room.

As the next wave of pressure and the ensuing pain came on,

there was only one answer to that kind of logic. I reached for the bottle.

The immediate sensation was one of burning around the nostrils where the skin was raw from having been constantly blown over the last few days. As I was recoiling from that, I experienced this revolting taste in the back of my throat immediately followed by. . . . . relief, smoothness and soothing. The throbbing in my head was gone, the incessant streaming eyes had gone, as was the burning in my ear, the intense pressure in my whole sinus area and my sore throat vanished. If I was to register the pain that I was experiencing on a one to ten level with ten being the peak, then I went from a ten to a two *in no more than three seconds.* I actually could not believe it. I could not understand what had happened having never experienced anything like this before. I was so astounded that I stayed lying down, convinced that at any moment the pain would come rushing back. Twenty minutes went by, nothing. By the time forty minutes had passed I was not only bored, I was feeling a complete idiot for the way in which I had behaved.

When I went back to bed for the night, I was still waiting for the pain to return but after an uninterrupted nights sleep, it was clearly not going to recur. The following morning there was a feeling like bruising in what had been the affected areas but that was to be expected as I still had the flu.

This was my introduction to Aloe Vera but even so I was not convinced and, I think, there were three reasons for this apparent ingratitude. The first was that, ironically, it was because the experience had been so quick, so effective and so inexplicable that I found myself doubting that it had really happened. The second is that we cannot store the physical experience of pain or discomfort and the further away from pain we get, the more vague the details. I was trying to convince myself that the injection had "kicked in" late, that maybe there had been a delayed reaction, at least this was a logical explanation. My instincts, however, told me otherwise. The third reason why I was not convinced was that I had not had such an experience before; if this third reason might seem a little weak then I would ask you to put yourself in a situation where you have the flu, with all the "add ons" that it brings you and then try to imagine squirting a juice of a plant up your nose and those very symptoms disappear in seconds. If you had no point of reference, how long would you maintain that it was the juice that had done it? By now, however, I was a curious cynic and it was on my next occasion of using Aloe Vera that I stopped needing a logical explanation and simply accepted that Aloe Vera does what it does, nothing more, nothing less.

For just over ten years, I had been suffering from a condition known as **Irritable Bowel Syndrome** or **I.B.S.** This can be debilitating to the point of hospitalisation. In my case it wasn't that bad but my symptoms were as though someone was wringing out my intestines, producing a cramping spasm, accompanied by a dull ache. This would strike at any time, without any warning and last for hours, if not days. Nothing had any effect, not changing my diet, massage, or even my trusty ol' hot water bottle. The doctor didn't know what caused it or what to suggest so I stopped seeing him after the first couple of years. My own belief is that it is caused by the accumulation of additives, pesticides, food colourings and flavourings that we add to our food. (I have no facts for this, call it a gut reaction!)

So one night as I was going to bed, I suddenly felt one of these spasms coming on. By this time, though, I had spoken to several people who also suffered from I.B.S. and they told me to take Aloe Vera juice. By now, we kept a bottle of juice in the fridge and so as the attack came on I drank four tablespoons of it and went to bed, fully expecting a night of painfully interrupted sleep.

Just as with the flu episode, what happened next was so contrary to anything that I had experienced, so quick and so "total" that it was difficult to take it in. As the Aloe Vera went down, the cramping relaxed, not just a little but completely. Areas that I didn't even know were tense unwound. Within minutes, my digestive system was making gurgling sounds similar to our heating system when the water first flows through the pipes! I felt this warming sensation as the Aloe Vera went on down, soothing as it went and as it soothed it took away the tension and as the tension went, so did the spasm and as the spasm went, so did I . . . . . into the best nights sleep for a decade.

Here was a condition for which there is no satisfactory remedy, that had dictated what I ate, my social life, my working life and my family life and which was tiring, not only physically but mentally too, (largely because of its unpredictability) and it was gone. Now, I eat what I like, have more energy and, as I complete my first year without an attack, the feeling of relief is as strong as ever. Somehow it seems appropriate that a condition which is not understood can be healed by a plant that is not understood! This time I was convinced, not only because of what I had experienced but, I believe, because I had a previous experience that I could relate it to. I.B.S. is a common condition that wrecks hundreds of thousands of lives. Imagine the effect it would have if this were to be their experience too.

So now that doubt was not an issue for me, my concern was more to do with what I considered to be a lack of information. I had been assured by fellow I.B.S. sufferers that Aloe Vera was perfectly safe to take and that it had no known side effects but I wanted to introduce Aloe Vera into my family's lifestyle and, with three children under five, I needed to be sure. There also appeared to be no guide as to how often, how much and in what form Aloe Vera should be used. (This is dealt with in Chapter 5 and Chapter 7ii). As I looked for this information, I began talking to people about Aloe Vera and the more I talked the more people wanted to try it. I was surprised at the amount of people who knew of it already; for some it was because on a holiday someone appeared with Aloe Vera leaves and relieved their sunburn or jelly fish sting immediately; others were aware of its ever increasing use in cosmetics and there were those who had an Aloe Vera plant or had a friend or relative who had a plant of their own that they had used for years as "the first aid" or "burn plant". The second thing that surprised me was not only the interest but also how fed up so many people are of "conventional" drugs.

Over the next few months, I had occasion to witness the effect that Aloe Vera had on family, friends, strangers and even pets. The changes that I saw were remarkable for different reasons, whether it was the rate at which healing took place or just because of the simplicity it didn't matter. What was astounding was the variety of different ailments that it could be used for. (See Chapter 7 i).There was the time when Fiona, my wife, had to stop drinking tea because it gave her abdominal pains. She started taking two spoonfuls of Aloe Vera in the morning and two in the evening and it went. This may sound nothing special but an ailment that had been bothering her for months cleared up *within forty eight hours*.

Then there was my mother-in-law, Pam. Pam runs a small farm and has a daily work rate that puts me to shame! However, just as her doctor had predicted, the lifestyle that she leads was literally starting to wear her out. Arthritis was creeping in and, by the beginning of this year it had got bad enough for the pain in her elbows to be waking her up every night. The drugs that she had been prescribed seemed to be doing nothing and it was getting to the stage where Pam was considering selling the farm (which is her life) as she would not be able to work it. After talking to her about Aloe Vera and its properties, she agreed to give it a try. A couple of weeks went by and nothing seemed to be happening. I felt terrible and could not understand why it wasn't working. I went to people who had had success with Aloe Vera and their arthritis. "Give it time" was the response and so Pam, to her credit, did.

It was about a week later that there were indications that something was starting to happen. The first was that Pam was starting to sleep through the night. Better rest added to the healing and after taking Aloe Vera for six weeks, she was out on the farm throwing bales of hay around! However, just as she was having success with her arthritis, Pam appeared at our cottage one day having had an accident.

She had been taking a cup of boiled milk out of her microwave when the cup slipped, spilling scalding milk all down her forearm, giving her second degree burns. As she was telling Fiona and I what had happened, she showed us the injury. I nearly threw up. (You may find the following description a little vivid but it is relevant.) About two thirds of the forearm was burnt. The burn was severe in two main areas which had come up as blisters each covering an area of about 5cms by 2.5cms. One of the blisters had burst leaving bits of skin hanging from the injury and the other was full of fluid and was raised to about 1cm. It was horrendous and Pam looked close to fainting.

Fortunately we had some Aloe Vera jelly and so Fiona covered a gauze in it and placed it gently on the injury. Pam immediately experienced relief from the pain and, Aloe Vera jelly in hand, she went home. This was on the Friday. The following day Fiona, the children and I dropped by Pam's farm to see how she was. Not only were we surprised to hear that Pam was "mucking out" the stables but, when we saw her, we were horrified to see that she had no dressing on the wound, which by this time had completely burst.

It was as Fiona was warming to the main theme of a spontaneous lecture about manure and its relation to infection that Pam stopped her in mid-flow (as she does!) saying "It's already getting better. I've been continually putting that jelly on the burn and there's no pain worth talking about. Look!" As we looked, it was clearly evident that, although it still looked pretty awful, the inflamed area had clearly reduced, there was no "gunge" just a light clean scab. There were no signs of excess fluid, weeping or infection. The damage had clearly been contained and was already on the mend.

The next time that I heard from Pam was on the Monday. She had been to the doctor to show her the injury. Apparently the doctor, who knew nothing about the accident until then, was surprised to see the advanced state of healing. She was also at a loss to understand how, considering Pam's muck chucking weekend, there was no sign of infection. Pam declined any of the medication that was offered and told the doctor that she had been using Aloe Vera. Why change when what she was already using worked?This produced a response that, sadly and frustratingly, is all too common and which was the catalyst for writing this book. The doctor immediately dismissed the whole incident. Despite having seen with her own eyes the extraordinary rate of healing, the doctor just shut down to the point of not returning my call to discuss what she had seen and how she might explain it.

None of this perturbed Pam in the least. Anyone and everyone that she came in contact with she told about this plant with these healing qualities. Got arthritis? Take Aloe Vera! Got eczema? Take Aloe Vera! Sore throat? Take Aloe Vera! Car engine seized? Take Aloe Vera! (Well almost!) She was a walking, talking commercial, The irony of it was that her arm was healing so fast that she was running out of promotion time! From the day of the accident to the day that I had to look long and hard to see the faintest of marks took just seventeen days. The doctor had said it would take over a month.

Then there were the results with the children. Tristan, one of my sons who is currently three and a half, has a fairly sensitive digestive system, with his tummy regularly experiencing bloating and diarrhoea. Without wishing to bore those of you who have not had children, walking around a supermarket with a child suffering from diarrhoea is only a fraction less stressful than walking around with a bomb packed around your waist, fitted with a mercury switch; the similarity being that either could go off at any time! Although this condition didn't bother Tristan, by the time he was three it was bothering me. On the next occasion that he was "afflicted" I gave him some Aloe Vera to drink. By the next time that he needed "to go" there was, shall we say, solid evidence that the Aloe Vera had worked! We kept him on Aloe Vera for a few weeks longer, by which time the flare ups had reduced greatly. Since then, there have been a number of changes that seemed to have started from this time. Not only is his tummy better but his appetite has improved. He sleeps much better, is consequently better rested and he has grown more consistently over the past six months. It is quite possible that Tristan has simply grown out of a particular phase. However his sustained accelerated growth along with the other changes signifies to me that his digestive process is functioning far better, enabling his body to benefit from this improved ability to absorb and process his food.

With the success of Tristan's tummy, there was one family member who needed it for the same reasons as Tristan, our dog, Roguey! After years of trying different foods and medications, the vet and I admitted defeat but I couldn't help but think that if it worked for people, why shouldn't it work for a dog? So I poured some Aloe Vera juice onto Roguey's food and

Presto! no more problems and no more vet bills! In addition a sore that Roguey had had on his nose for about six months healed up too.

These are only some of the successes that I and my family have had with Aloe Vera. I could continue with how it has alleviated sunburn, nettle stings, insect bites and stings, nappy rash, razor burn and bleeding gums but I have possibly overdone it already and there are many more examples from many different people included in the rest of the book.

I mentioned in the introduction that the main problem that I had was one of (in)credibility. Maybe you can understand why. For those of you who are finding this a little far fetched, I quite understand. I would, however, like you to consider a line of thought that may challenge your own current way of thinking.

When you go to the doctor and are given a prescription, what do you know about it? If you are told what the chemical make-up of that drug is, does it mean anything to you? Do you know what side effects it may have? Does it have any long term effects? Does your doctor know? Might your doctor have got the information from the sales representative of the company that made the drug? How long do drugs companies test their products for before releasing them on the market? Have you heard of a drugs company having to withdraw a product because it wasn't safe?

Alternatively, if your doctor were to tell you that you were to take a product which has been used in medicine longer than any other known "treatment", that it was known to be safe, non toxic and totally natural with no side effects and an excellent result factor, would you take it?

For those who think that these questions are alarmist, there is a group of doctors, who do not wish to be named, who believe that within the U.K. health service as many as 1 in 10 hospital medical beds are occupied by iatrogenic cases. Iatrogenic means "induced unintentionally by a physician's treatment." In other words, side effects or combined effects from various drugs treatments. In other words, an unwanted effect from a combination of drugs.

CHAPTER 2

ALOE VERA, DESCRIPTION & ORIGIN

When I first saw an Aloe Vera plant I thought it was a cactus, (see cover) and so was surprised to hear, that along with over 200 other different types of Aloe, it is a member of the lily family. The word is a derivative from the Arabic word "alloeh" meaning shining, bitter substance, (I'm sure those who have tried it will agree!) The species name (ie. which Aloe is which) differs. The aloe that this book is dealing with is known as Aloe Barbadensis, or Aloe Vera, meaning true aloe, (in this book it will referred to as Aloe Vera.) It is important to note that different Aloes contain different properties.

The Aloe grouping also belongs to a larger family known as Xeroids. What is particular to this family is their ability to "shut down" their stomata (or pores) thus preventing water loss, enabling the plant to survive periods of drought. In addition, almost all Xeroids have a process which closes off any damaged area almost immediately, again preventing water loss. Once the wound is healed over, the plant continues growing from the damaged point but in a different direction.

Aloe Vera, as I mentioned, looks like it could be a cactus and with Aloes ranging in size from as little as one inch in height to a tree like fifty feet, a mature Aloe Vera will average about two and a half feet. The leaves will make up almost all of this height as the stem hardly emerges above the ground. As the leaves grow upward, ending in a point, they are covered in a green, thick skin that is almost rubbery in texture, along the sides of which are barbs. From side to side the leaf has a curve that is similar to rhubarb and celery and the formation of the leaves I understand is called a rosette pattern. (If there is any-one who, like me, doesn't quite get this description, then the leaves on top of a pineapple grow in a rosette formation!) It is within these leaves that a thick fillet of clear jelly is produced and it is this jelly that contains the variety of healing properties that are unique to this plant, ranging from antibiotic, coagulat-ing (ie clotting) agent, pain killing and growth stimulating.

Thanks to paintings of Aloe on the walls of the temples and tombs of ancient Egypt, we can date the first signs of man's relationship with Aloe to around 4,000 B.C. with the first writ-ten account of its use at around 1750-1500 B.C. It would appear that all the ancient and great civilisations and empires of the world used Aloe. In addition to the Egyptians, the Greeks, Romans, Persians, Indians and Chinese used this plant in their medical practice, the Greeks and Romans in particular keeping records as to its value.

Historians tell of Alexander the Great being advised by Aristotle to capture an island called Socotra, not because of any particular strategic value but because the island's industry was Aloe farming. The island was duly taken and the Greeks went on their way with Aloe growing in the wagons that fol-lowed behind. This way, there was a fresh supply of Aloe on hand for the treating of wounds. I like this story not only for its ingenuity but as a great commercial for Aloe. Not did only one of the finest minds the world has ever known endorse the prod-uct but I can't believe that "Big Al'" would take time out of a hectic "conquering the known world" schedule for anything that wasn't of great benefit to him or his troops!

Aloe is also mentioned in the Bible. After the crucifixion of Christ, Nichodemis took a mixture of myrrh and aloes to the burial chamber:-

John 19: 39-40.
39. And there came also Nichodemis which at first came
to Jesus by night and brought a mixture of myrrh and
aloes about an hundred pound weight.

40.Then they took the body of Jesus and wound it in
linen cloths with spices as the manner of the Jews is to
bury.

Through the centuries Aloe spread throughout the world. As trade increased amongst countries and then continents so Aloe seemed to appear. Both Marco Polo and Columbus's voyages witnessed and logged the spread of the plant. Aloe outlasted many empires that introduced the plant to their new and conquered lands. The empires may have collapsed but the plant remained.

Aloe literally came under the microscope of modern medicine in the 1930's. At this time x-ray technology was new and on occasions a hit or miss affair. Patients suffering from radiation burns and ulcers were not responding to medication. No modern drug could be found to have any effect on this modern invention and yet in the U.S.A. Aloe began to be used and was found to be most effective. With the invention of the atomic bomb there was a more sinister "need to know". Examination of survivors from the Hiroshima and Nagasaki bombs treated with Aloe Vera, revealed seemingly inexplicable healing, tissue growth and reduced pain and scarring *where all other therapeutic attempts had failed.*

By this time research had largely been carried out both in the (then) Soviet Union and the U.S.A. and no matter how hard the plant was studied, there were two consistent factors that seemed unsolvable the first of which was no one could find out how Aloe Vera works. To this day the plant refuses to yield its secret, although over the years it has certainly revealed its main constituents. The second factor that had seemed unsolvable was the problem of oxidising. When a fresh Aloe is opened, it will immediately begin to oxidise which leads to a reduction in potency. Refrigeration helps but only in slowing the process. In 1964 a practising pharmacist by the name of

Bill Coats was determined to find a way to somehow stabilise this reaction, thus making it possible to process the plant, making it available to anyone, anywhere.

In 1968, Mr. Coats succeeded. The juice he began producing maintained the properties previously only found in a fresh leaf of Aloe and consequently thousands upon thousands of people have experienced relief where before they had pain, suffering and often misery.

As just one of those who has benefited in so many ways, I would like to extend a huge personal thanks to Mr. Coats for all his effort.

CHAPTER 3

ALOE VERA, WHAT IT IS & WHAT IT DOES

One of the problems that I had when I started to find out more about Aloe Vera was that when I asked what was in it and I was told that there were all sorts of vitamins, amino acids, minerals etc., it didn't actually help because although I was familiar with the terms, I didn't know what they were or what they did or how they help us. As far as I was aware, coal was a mineral and should I be taking anything with the word "acid" in it? There was a certain sense of relief as I asked around to discover that I wasn't the only one feeling a bit of a fool at not knowing these things and so I was fortunate to hear that there was a doctor who was trying out Aloe Vera on his patients. His name is Dr. Peter Atherton and he kindly answered any questions that I had.

My thanks to Peter who, having been briefed by me to use only short and simple words, went through the agonising process of waiting for some sign, however vague, that could be taken to mean that I was finally grasping the most basic of medical concepts. In chapter 5 he talks about Aloe Vera and how he tested his patients, this section is about how his patience was tested!

What I first wanted to know was what is in Aloe Vera and what effects these ingredients have on people?

The constituents that make up Aloe Vera:

1) **Vitamins A, B1, B2, B6, B12, C & E**. . . . . . vitamins can be defined as being a small part of the diet necessary for proper growth and maintenance of health. They are different from all other areas of the diet in their structure, potency and effect. Vitamins cannot be manufactured within the body and some cannot be stored, so it is necessary for the diet to sustain a continuous supply. Some vitamins, (A&D in particular) can be harmful if there is too much in the system. Conversely, it is just possible to survive without them, although it would not be in a state of good health as the individual would be prone to disease and infection, therefore shortening life expectancy. What do these individual vitamins do?:-

Vitamin A (Retinol) is essential for night vision. Deficiency can lead to night blindness, skin and membrane hardening and defective dentition.

Vitamin B is grouped together for no other reason than that they are all water soluble. Deficiency of this group as a whole can lead to beriberi.

Vitamin B1, (Thiamine) is essential for the health of nerve tissue and the functioning of the cardiac and gastrointestinal systems. Lack of B1 leads to irritability, energy loss and anorexia.

Vitamin B2 (Riboflavin) helps generate healthy skin and membrane tissue.

Vitamin B6 (Pyridoxine) assists growth.

Vitamin B12 is present almost exclusively in dairy and meat produce as well as eggs. To find it present in a plant is rare and therefore of great relevance to vegans.

Lack of vitamin B12 can lead to anaemia and neuropathy. (Neuropathy is a disease or disfunction of the nerves, typically causing numbness and weakness.) B12 is also used in conjunction with other vitamins for premenstrual tension and associated depression.

Vitamin C (Ascorbic acid) was long ago known to prevent scurvy. Nowadays it is commonly associated with cold and flu prevention. In addition, it is needed as part of the formation of tissue fibres, therefore the lack of it could be felt severely.

Vitamin E (tocopherol) although identified some time ago was incorrectly thought to have possible fertility implications. In more recent times its role in the area of skin health and tissue growth was recognised, with some also saying that it is capable of helping to fight infection and respiratory disorders.

2) **Minerals: Calcium, chromium, copper, magnesium, manganese, zinc, sodium chloride, potassium,** ....
   .. The body contains approximately twenty major minerals all of which must be derived from food. Minerals are required for three main purposes: a) as constituents of bones; notably calcium, phosphorous and magnesium. b) As constituents of the cells of the body; notably iron, phosphorous, sulphur and potassium. c) As soluble salts giving the fluids of the body the balance and stability essential to life; in particular, sodium, chlorine, calcium and potassium. Minerals can be harmful if the body contains too much or too little of them.

Calcium is the most abundant mineral in the body and is the chief material of bones and teeth. It also regulates the fluids in the body and enhances communication in the nervous system, allowing the body to work as it should, maintaining optimum response of muscle to nervous stimulation. It is also a key player in normal clotting of the blood, (eg. when there is a cut or graze.)

Calcium is absorbed in the upper part of the small intestine. Deficiency results in rickets and reduced growth in children.

Chromium promotes enzyme activity. (See enzyme.)

Copper is used in the formation of blood.

Magnesium plays a vital part in the metabolism of the body. The importance of magnesium can be judged by the fact that lack of it can lead to convulsions and even death.

Manganese, like magnesium, is noticeable when missing, resulting in slower growth, nervous disorders and infertility. It is found in enzyme and amino acid activity and is involved in the process of releasing energy from food.(See enzyme and amino acid.)

Zinc is also noticed in its absence, possibly bringing on anaemia. However, high contents of zinc found in that well known aphrodisiac the oyster, have raised questions about its role in that field!

Sodium chloride is essential to ensure a sufficient alkaline environment for certain digestive enzymes to function. It is critical for keeping a normal water balance in the body. Together with potassium it can be called one of the regulators of the body.

Potassium, as has been said, regulates except that its "domain" is in the muscle cells and blood plasma (the fluid component of blood,) helping muscle action and water retention.

Although this is an understandable explanation of the minerals themselves it does not explain what these "amino acids", "enzymes" and "proteins" do.

Amino acids, of which there are seventeen in Aloe Vera, are required in the body because it takes hundreds of them to make one molecule of protein.

Protein is essential to all living matter. It is mainly used in the structural formation of tissue, with any surplus being used for (heat making) fuel/energy.

Enzymes are a catalyst for chemical reaction, change and breakdown. Every time you put food in your mouth, it is the enzymes that immediately get to work on breaking it down, without they themselves changing form in any way. There must be thousands of enzymes as each has its own particular task. The well being of any individual depends greatly on changes that take place within them and, therefore, on the enzymes that it can produce. All enzymes, by the way, are protein.

The next, and final, three constituents of Aloe Vera I had never previously heard of :

Saponins form foam in water solution and are used as detergents and emulsifiers. They have natural cleansing and antiseptic qualities.

Lignin is a "wood-like" pulp. It has the ability to penetrate the skin.

Anthraquinones of which there are fourteen present in Aloe Vera, have antibiotic, antiviral, antibacterial and anti-inflammatory properties. They also stimulate the bowel, and have an enzyme-like action, in the way they remove dead tissue and have certain pain killing properties.

This is the list of ingredients that make up about 5% of Aloe Vera. The other 95% being water. So, if you put this extraordinary combination into your body, how might it benefit you?

CHAPTER 4

THE HEALING PROPERTIES OF ALOE VERA

This chapter is partially based on a presentation made by a chiropractic doctor from America, a Dr.Gregg Henderson, who has used Aloe Vera extensively in his practise for over twelve years.The healing properties of Aloe Vera can be witnessed and experienced but not fully explained. As such, the following are properties that have been witnessed time after time, after time:

1) Anti-inflammatory:-

To explain anti-inflammatory, it would make sense to understand what inflammation is. The body responds to injury like wounding or a burn, with inflammation. This consists of heat, swelling, redness and pain. The redness is due to the increase of blood to the damage area. Normally, the capillaries (the smallest blood vessel) allow the exchange of water and small molecules between tissue and blood. When inflamed, bigger protein molecules "get through" causing increased pressure on the walls of the capillaries, resulting in swelling. It used to be thought of that the heat generated in inflammation was a "byproduct". This is not the case, it is the increase activity and flow of the blood. The raise in temperature will therefore only be close to that of an individual's blood. The pain is caused partly by the pressure of the swelling, partly from nerve damage.

Inflammation is one of the major areas that doctors have to fight. In diseases such as arthritis, the only aspect that is really understood is the inflammation process not the disease. Normally, a disease such as rheumatoid arthritis would be treated with anti-inflammatory drugs and steroids, (cortisone), which has been said to have the effect of "putting out the fire but does nothing to take care of the fire damage" and in addition there are many negative side effects that are associated with long term use, e.g. weight increase, thinning and bruising of the skin, osteoporosis. (Osteoporosis causes fragile/brittle bones.) However, **Aloe Vera has a steroid like action** with two major advantages. The first is that there are no side effects and the second is that it not only puts out the fire but it takes care of the damage better than any conventional drug that I have seen. Part of this "damage relief" comes, particularly when inflammation becomes infected. Aloe Vera has what Dr. Henderson refers to as **"The Lecithin Like Ingredient"**. Lecithin actually means emulsify which is when you have two liquids that are dispersed throughout each other in small droplets. In the case of infection it goes through this emulsifying process which, in turn, stimulates the liver and kidneys which obligingly then remove the waste.

Dr. Henderson quotes a colleague who has reduced healing cycles down from 6 weeks to 1 week and from 1 week to 1 day, since using Aloe Vera, largely due to the fact that Aloe Vera reduces inflammation and suppresses bacteria and therefore infection.

Aloe Vera is **antibiotic, virucidal and bactericidal**. It actually suppresses the growth of bacteria *and has even been found effective against typhoid*, one of the toughest strains. In addition it is **antipuritic**, relieves itching, **antipyritic** relieves heat and fungicidal killing a range of fungus infections.

It is **Keratolytic** (ie. destroys/softens hard skin.) Aloe is **deep penetrating**, taking down its healing properties to the damaged area. It then strips the toxic materials, increases blood circulation to the area and flushes the dead tissue away.

In addition the enzymes in Aloe Vera break down the fatty layers and replace them with water, providing a healthier environment to further the healing process.

Growth Stimulator

There is little official recognition about any of Aloe Vera's qualities. However, the F.D.A. (Federal Drugs Authority) in the U.S.A. agrees that Aloe Vera has properties that enhance the regeneration of new tissue, resulting in an **accelerated rate of healing**. Hospitals have experienced **50% better results** in the treatment of burns and significant improvement in the after effects of **radiation effects on cancer treatment**. Leg ulcers, common amongst diabetics, sometimes never heal with conventional medicine. With Aloe Vera they have been healed in weeks.

Aloe Vera **moisturises** without closing off oxygen, which is crucial to the healing process and as it does so it replaces the fluids lost that are needed to heal. This could be why it **reduces scarring**.

To conclude, the **proliferation of cells** is, of course growth stimulation. As the Aloe Vera removes dead tissues it increases the circulation and therefore the supply of nutrition. This reduces scabbing and therefore scarring, increasing moisture and therefore revitalisation, giving tissue what it needs.

You only get good results if you have good tissue. Aloe Vera revitalises good tissue and it makes the tissue function better from the cellular level.

DETOXIFICATION: If you can't get rid of the toxins or waste, the tissue will not have the ability to heal properly. In detoxification, one of the main objectives is the increased ability to get rid of waste. Potassium, found in Aloe Vera, stimulates the kidneys to get rid of the waste.

When you take something into your mouth, it is mixed with enzymes to start the digestive process. It goes into the stomach and is then pushed out into the small intestine. As it goes into the intestinal area different nutrients are absorbed in different areas. The wall of the intestine is similar to fingers on a hand and as food moves through the intestine, (as it does down a snake,) these fingers are there to absorb what they can from the food. However these fingers have cells packed around them, which, in turn, have "micro fingers" packed around them, and it is here that the absorbing takes place. These little cells fall off and rejuvenate all the time.

However it is not only the nutrients from the food that are absorbed, it is the sludge too. It is no secret that the food we eat is covered in chemicals, insecticides, additives, saturated fats etc. and it is because of all this rubbish that intestinal problems in the U.S.A. and the U.K. in particular, have soared. Because all this sludge blocks up the cells, slowing the system down, these cells then have little ability to absorb anything and so absorption is reduced. Remember, different nutrients are absorbed in different areas. This shows potentially how quickly we can become nutritionally deficient. In a short period of time the cells end up being packed, drowning in slime and junk which begins to putrefy. It can't be absorbed, it can't be eliminated, so it sits and rots. This is when the bowel problems really set in and where Aloe Vera is at its most impressive. A classic bowel problem is ulcers of different types. Dr. Henderson's clinic has people coming in, scheduled for surgery on stomach ulcers the next week. They are given a tablespoon an hour to flush the system through. Dr. Henderson has *never* had a case go to surgery with the many, many ulcer cases that he has treated either greatly reduced or completely healed.

Aloe Vera is used in both **chronic diarrhoea** *and* **chronic constipation**. What is diarrhoea? It is the body trying to get rid of its bowel content because it can't process it. It has an **inflamed bowel**. Aloe Vera not only bathes the tissue but it softens and moisturises the layer of sludge and cleans out the intestine. By complete contrast, Dr. Henderson treats sufferers of chronic constipation, individuals who may excrete nothing for **two weeks** and when they finally do, they produce what looks like rabbit pellets and yet they are eating normally. All this food is being absorbed but only to a certain degree, when it becomes indigestible, hard, dehydrated lumps. It is actually possible to feel the lumps. Aloe Vera loosens up the area, increases absorption, increases elimination and restarts the regenerative process.

Dr. Henderson concludes: if you can absorb Aloe Vera then you get **increased regeneration**. Once your regeneration process is increased then you get better absorption of nutrition and body function, which leads to **better assimilation/processing**. In other words, if your intestine is clean, it will give better nutrition from the food that you eat. **Better nutrition** makes you feel better, the tissues work better and better function **at the cellular level. Better functioning throughout gives more energy**.

Because of the "instant" society where we use colouring, dyes, insecticides etc. that we know are bad for us, detoxification is important as a regular aspect of our lives. (When I see people working out, I wonder whether they realise that if they got the inside of their body as fit as the outside they would feel even better and their work out would probably be easier too.) Aloe Vera plays an important part not only in a nutritional aspect but in eliminating and competing with those aspects of our society that are not good for us.

We continually hear of the miracle of Aloe Vera. The miracle of Aloe Vera is that it makes tissue function better <u>at the cellular level.</u> If the cell is better, the body is better and if the body is better then our quality of life is better . . . . . and that is the benefit that Aloe Vera can give all of us.

CHAPTER 5

DR. PETER ATHERTON

Dr. Atherton, M.B. ChB. D.Obst. R.C.O.G. M.R.C.G.P. is a rare and valuable species in the world of Aloe Vera. He is rare because he is a "conventional" doctor who, despite his initial cynicism, was prepared to read about and personally try Aloe Vera in order that he could form his own opinion. He is valuable for two reasons, the first of which is that, having been impressed by the effect Aloe Vera had on him personally, Dr. Atherton then decided to try it out on some of his patients, (at the time of writing this, the number is forty.) The second reason is that "conventional" medicine is being challenged and questioned in a manner that has never been experienced by the profession before. It is having to account for itself and its attitude and it is having to change. Dr. Atherton represents that change and the new approach for which I applaud him.

Before going into specifics about his group of patients, there were a few questions that I am regularly asked that Dr. Atherton gave me his personal view point on. For instance, taking Aloe Vera with medication he regards as fine as he knows of no interactions with plant juice and drugs. With regards to any side effects, he will never say no-one will have side effects because there may always be one element to which one individual may be allergic. However, *generally* the answer to whether there are side effects has to be "no". As to dosage, Dr. Atherton recommends between one and four fluid ounces a day. If diarrhoea or colic like pains persist for more than 2-3 days then reduce the dose. As to how quickly it will take effect, for some it is instant, others months. It depends on the individual and the problem.

About the trials: Before continuing with the details of the trials it must be noted that they have been going on for a short period of time, (just over two months in the longest case) and are still ongoing. Dr. Atherton is only speaking in general terms at the moment. In 1995 there will be a book produced between us on the full progress and results of these trials.

Selecting the group:

In selecting the patients who were to try Aloe Vera, Dr. Atherton had three criteria:

1) That the condition had to be chronic.

2) That they must have had standard medical treatment to not much or no effect. (They had all either been treated for months or years.)

3) They had to fall in one of three groups, dermatological, bowel, other. Those that are in the dermatological group are suffering from psoriasis, eczema, ulcers, urticaria. (Urticaria is an allergic reaction that is similar in its manifestation to nettle rash. Severe cases require treatment with adrenaline of corticosteroids.) Those in the bowel group are suffering from Irritable Bowel Syndrome (I.B.S.) Diverticulitis and Colitis. Those in the "other" group range from M.E. non-specific rheumatism, arthritis and asthma.

Feed back: The overwhelming feed back from the vast majority of cases reported an aspect that had not been considered. Although not all the symptoms had cleared up, the patients reported a clear sense of well being, saying they felt better, happier, had more energy and were sleeping better.

This feedback was particularly relevant with the M.E. sufferers whose main problem is a lack of energy and "well being".

In 90% of the patients (ie. 36 out of the 40 patients) the symptoms improved from slightly to dramatically. These were people who had chronic conditions that had failed to respond to months or years of "conventional" treatment.

Think of the number of people who go to their doctor for help with the conditions that are listed in this trial. Then think of the effect on our health services, the costs that it would save, if the number you thought of was also reduced by 90%.

I mentioned that Dr. Atherton and I are putting together a book on the results of the trials that are being conducted. If you or anyone you know would like to take part, then would you write to me c/o The Wordsmith Publishing Company. We are always looking for people, not necessarily only for those groups listed.

CHAPTER 6
TESTIMONIALS

Introduction: The following letters that you are about to read are from individuals who have used Aloe Vera based products and had such positive results that they wrote to the people who introduced them to Aloe Vera. Consequently, there are references to Forever Living Products, or F.L.P. which is the largest producer of Aloe Vera in the world. In addition, there are products like deep heat and propolis cream mentioned which are part of the F.L.P. range of Aloe Vera based products. These letters have all been written completely voluntarily, coming from a feeling of relief and gratitude. I have abbreviated some in order to keep to the point, on all I have reduced names to initials. Should there be anyone that you would like to write to, then please contact me c/o Wordsmith Publishing Company and I'll see what can be arranged. I am indebted to these people who selflessly gave testimony to the healing qualities of Aloe Vera.

ARTHRITIS:

Dear Rodney,

When you first introduced Aloe Vera Juice to me your words were that you "couldn't promise a miracle cure." Having suffered with arthritis in my right knee for 2 years or more and gradually worsening I had tried many things but resigned myself to soon be needing sticks to help me.

I have had just one litre of Aloe Vera Juice and the change is remarkable. I can outwalk friends and on a recent holiday in Corfu I walked many miles. I can now resume my dancing which my wife and I enjoy very much and even run upstairs despite my soon reaching the age of 70 with Bronchial problems.

So Rodney it may not be a miracle cure for some but it certainly has been a blessing for me.

Many thanks,

Yours sincerely,

John D. (Leeds. U.K.) 08:12:92

ARTHRITIS:

Dear John and Joanne Stokes,
I am writing to thank you for introducing me to Aloe Vera Gel, it has certainly made a big difference to my life.
As you know I have been suffering with arthritis in my spine, neck and shoulders for the past two and a half years, which set in after an accident at work.
Although it was difficult for me to accept the restrictions and affects the condition was having on my life at first, I learned to pace myself, so that I didn't tackle too many house-hold chores in one day, I gave up gardening which I loved so much, and reading or doing a crossword with my head bent forward for long periods, was out of the question, because it caused me so much pain and discomfort.
By the time I met you both I had undergone physiotherapy treatment, acupuncture, traction and steroid

injection in my upper spine to relieve pain from a trapped nerve, I was fast running out of treatments to get some relief.

I was also taking some very strong aspirin based tablets, which upset my stomach, consequently I had to take other drugs to line the stomach first. Much as I hated taking all these drugs, I needed them to keep the inflammation under control.

It really was my lucky day when you introduced me to Forever Living Products, and especially the Aloe Vera Gel, because I no longer take all those drugs. I take 2oz every morning and it really does the trick. Life is worth living again.

Thankyou for the miracle of Aloe.

Regards June W.(East Hunsbury, Northampton, U.K.) 17:07:94

Dear John,

I have suffered from arthritis and glandular fever for a number of years, often causing depression. Since using Aloe Vera juice, the arthritis has practically gone, and any lethargy and tiredness caused by the fever have also disappeared.

The best form of medication I have found for these problems.

Yours sincerely,

David. A. C. (Earls Croome, Worcs, U.K.) 26:06:94

ARTHRITIS:

Dear Sir,

I have Rheumatoid Arthritis. In 1985 I was a very sick woman, I was just 5 stone 10oz, all I did was lay in bed all the time, even the doctors could do no more, I was

taking all different kinds of medicine and tablets, but nothing I took made any difference. Then along came Caroline Headington with Aloe Vera, I thought well I will give it a try, I can't lose anything by it. I started taking three sherry glasses full every day for quite a long time, then I began to feel a lot better. I felt as though I wanted to get up out of bed and get dressed which I did and come down stairs. Of course all my clothes were too big for me as I was so thin I only took a size eight. Well as I grew stronger and put on weight, I reduced the dose to two glasses a day. Caroline was marvellous I had the gel also from her to rub in any pains I had especially in my arms, which also worked. Caroline would come and see me to make sure I was alright. To cut a long story short I am now wearing a size 16, I am about 10st 5oz. Without Carolyn's and of course Aloe Vera's help I don't think that I would have survived, now I take one sherry glass a day which I could not do without.........I have nothing but praise for Carolyn and Aloe Vera
I (have) still got the arthritis but not as bad as I had it, I feel much better and its a treat to be alive, without Aloe Vera and the help of Caroline I don't think that it would have been possible.
Yours,

Valerie G.(Pontypool, Gwent, U.K.)

Dear John,
I have had arthritis for quite a few years and after sitting down for a few hours, found it difficult to walk. Since taking Aloe Vera I find that a lot of the aches are gone and it is a lot easier to walk.
yours faithfully,
H.C.L. (Worcester,U.K.) 08:07:94

ARTHRITIS:

Dear Rex,
I must admit that the aloe vera gel drink has done my arthritis a power of good because now I can go ten days at a time without pain or any kind of swelling to my legs and back. At one time I couldn't write a letter because I couldn't hold a pen for more than 45 seconds, which was really painful so I must say thankyou for your wonderful product, its a world beater, there's nothing to match it anywhere.
I'm sure that if it wasn't for the aloe vera drink I wouldn't be walking now, I'd be stuck in a wheelchair instead. I now know that it is wonderful to feel alive again.
Yours sincerely,
Rob D. (Birmingham, U.K.)

Dear Sir/Madam,
I am looking for a local supplier of your Aloe Vera Tonic. . .
I am interested partly for me but mainly for an arthritic goat of mine who I'd rather not put down but the vets can do nothing for her and my mother says that this tonic has so completely cured her arthritis that even her doctor can find no evidence of it now.
Please help me - urgently - if you can.
Sincerely,
C.S.(Helston, Cornwall,U.K.)

BOWEL:

I had a serious bowel operation 15 years ago which necessitated me having to have 7 feet of my bowel intestines removed. This left me with a constant dose of diarrhoea, which was embarrassing and most uncomfortable, especially while visiting, travelling or on social occasions. I actually dreaded travelling and was virtually a prisoner in my own home. I have been to several *doctors, attended numerous clinics and I am virtually a medical guinea pig, but all to no avail. I had to go on a strict diet which strictly limited my intake of varieties in food. No beef and root vegetables were allowed. Since I started taking Aloe Vera Gel approximately three times daily my bowel complaint has improved immensely within **a day** of taking the gel.*

In the last week I have eaten beef, lettuce and cabbage, food that I thought I'd never eat again, and my bowel has in that short time become regular. I would strongly recommend also the heat lotion which cured my aching neck which was very stiff. I got instant relief on just one application of the rub. I would strongly recommend it to my friends.

Bridget R.

IRRITABLE BOWEL SYNDROME:

I have had problems with what the Doctors have described as an irritated bowel since May, 1991. The symptoms were a "migraine" type pain in the stomach, loss of appetite, lack of energy and disturbed sleep. I have tried conventional medication, and have had exploratory surgery with no real success. I also tried reflexology and found that to be of some benefit.

I was introduced to Forever Living Products in June. I have used Forever Living Aloe Vera Gel (which is actually a juice) and also Bee Pollen Tablets. Within six weeks I have found, the frequency and severity of these attacks have reduced by half. Lack of energy is no longer a problem, I feel more relaxed and my sleep pattern has improved. I would highly recommend these products.

Michael B.

BOWEL: COLITIS

I had suffered from Colitis for over a year. The symptoms I had were acute pain every morning followed by the necessity to dash to the toilet. I had diarrhoea and constant niggly pains throughout each day and bleeding also. My lifestyle was very restricted as the maximum time I could go out for was two hours, general and social activities were very difficult. Life was very restricted and worrying for me. I had put off going to the doctors as two friends of mine who also suffered from Colitis had little or no relief from the medications they were prescribed, and their lifestyles were very much restricted also. I was hoping it might just get better but the symptoms became much worse and I couldn't cope much longer without some help.

I was very skeptical but my daughter whose family are completely convinced of the benefits of using Aloe Vera persuaded me to try it for myself and assured me that it certainly wouldn't do me any harm or make me any worse than I was, so I reluctantly agreed to try it. She suggested I drink 1 fl.oz. 3 x daily to clear my system very quickly. It was most definitely effective at clearing ... I felt it was too effective at clearing me out ... I already suffered from diarrhoea and taking the Gel I felt the need to use the toilet even more frequently.

She suggested it would be better to bear the frequency for a week or so until it settled down, she felt a faster detoxification would save me from having to endure all my symptoms for a longer time. However I felt more comfortable about a slower detoxification and decided to reduce the quantities. After three weeks of taking 1fl.oz. per day, sipped at intervals, I began to receive some very positive results. The bleeding and diarrhoea was intermittent and not so frequent, the pain was gone.

I drank a total of three (one litre) bottles over a three month period, and by that time all my symptoms were gone! I was very happy. My daughter felt that if I had taken the suggested amounts I would have had all the results much sooner, but whatever, I was still very much relieved to be rid of all the unpleasantries.

About two or three months later I had a slight remission but in no way as severe as I had prior to first taking Aloe

Vera. I immediately requested a couple more bottles of Aloe Vera which I drank over a two month period. The symptoms quickly vanished and since that time in 1992 I have not needed to request any more. I have been given a couple of bottles each time my son-in-law and daughter visit us a couple of times a year, as I firmly believe that prevention is better than cure and I know that it has completely enabled me to lead a normal and very active lifestyle once more. Forever Living Products don't claim that Aloe Vera is very effective however I would recommend to anyone to try.

I was such a skeptic, about using Aloe Vera before, I wish I had started using it earlier. I would be happy to talk to anyone about it.

Jean.M.W.

BOWEL: CROHN'S DISEASE

I was diagnosed as having Crohn's Disease in 1984. To anyone who may not know, Crohn's disease is a severe disorder of the stomach and bowel. For me it was the cause of bouts of severe diarrhoea and stomach cramping that rendered me disabled in the sense, I was unable to work or function properly on a daily basis. My social and working life had to be planned or re-organised daily depending on my condition that day.

Serious attempts at diet change over eight years failed to help in any way. Theses changes varied from including or excluding "root vegetable", "greens", "roughage", "starch", "alcohol", and "common beverages", etc. Time passed with two operations and several changes of medication all, while they worked for a short period, in the long run brought their own problems, thus worsening my condition.

Left in a "medical limbo", I turned to Forever Living Products, Aloe Berry Nectar as a skeptic who said, with a 60-day Money Back Guarantee, I had nothing to lose. I would now without hesitation, recommend it to anyone who would to like to try a natural answer to their health problems. Wishing you whoever you may be all the best.

Gerard R.

IRRITABLE BOWEL SYNDROME:

In December 1993, after suffering from I.B.S. (Irritable Bowel Syndrome) for over 8 years, I discovered a purely natural product that, unlike many "treatments" I had tried, seemed to be helping me.

The product is Forever Living Products pure Aloe Vera gel.

To give you an idea of the effect the Aloe has had, I'll explain what living with I.B.S. has been like. From what I remember I seemed to start suffering from I.B.S. after working for some time doing shift work. I have discovered from talking to other I.B.S. sufferers, that some of them have also experienced this.

The causes and effects of I.B.S. varies from individual to individual. I personally react badly to alcohol, spicy food, rich sauces and citric fruits, made all the worse if I feel under stress. The effect the above have on me is severe distension of the gut, causing a lot of internal pressure, and consequently in some situation, extreme pain. From this I will suffer either bad constipation or diarrhoea, each causing as much discomfort as the other.

I have tried Fibregel, peppermint oil capsules and Colofac (a drug to help with bowel spasms), from my doctor which never seemed to have much effect. But to be totally honest, I found too much of a hassle to take, and personally hated the Fibregel.

I spent extra money going to a homeopathic doctor, who's "diet" definitely seemed to help, however after nearly two months of not being able to touch alcohol, spicy foods and other enjoyable food & drink, I couldn't stand it any more!

I believe that because of the nature of I.B.S., if the "medication", "treatment" taken isn't convenient or restricts your eating pleasures, it is unlikely that you will stay with that programme long term.

What I have experienced with Forever Living Products

Aloe Vera Gel, despite the fact it doesn't taste too great, is it is convenient and most importantly I can enjoy the food and drink that upset me so badly.

I take about two tablespoons full, morning and evening, and I have experienced a huge difference in the way I feel. I cannot say at this moment in time after just 3 months that it has healed, as I occasionally will still suffer, but to a much lesser degree.

However, if I progress at the rate I am, I feel very confident that after maybe 12 to 18 months, I may be able to say I no longer suffer from I.B.S.!!

If you would like to know any more about the Aloe Vera gel and Irritable Bowel Syndrome feel free to call me, I'd be more than happy to help.

Regards,
Alison C. (London.)

BURNS:

Dear Pam,

The day you recommended to me Aloe Gelly for the treatment of the burns that I had received to my feet was a turning point in my life.

Many years ago, in 1981, whilst building a wall at the bottom of my garden which has a brook running by. My feet came into contact with the concrete I was using for the base. Unknown to me at the time the concrete had a very high lime content to enable it to dry in the wet condition. The lime had burnt through the Wellington boots that I was wearing and created ulcers to the ankle and lower parts of my feet. My doctor at that time was unsure what to do. After some considerable time the doctor became aware of the fact that she had not prescribed the right treatment and as time went on my feet became ulcerated and very painful. The situation arose where it was very likely that I would have to have skin-grafts. However, at last, due to being sent to the special burns unit at Aylesbury I received excellent treatment and over a long period the surface burns healed. I was left with scarred ankles. I suffered a great deal of pain for many years due to the fact that I now had only one layer of skin protecting the ankle areas.

I had great difficulty walking in the mornings on arising from bed and the minutest knock would create ulcers. The worst was to come; very frequently my legs would burn internally, which at times was unbearable. The only real relief I had was to soak some bandages and put them in the freezer and use them when they were frozen.

I have been prescribed many products, none of which have worked. I used Aloe Gelly and within 48 hours I was experiencing relief that I hadn't known for many years. To this day I have no real pain or discomfort.

The only problem I have experienced is the after effects; my nails have begun to grow quicker and stronger.

I would like to say to you "thanks" and to FLP I will always be grateful.

M.D.H. 18th Jan.'94. (Milton Keynes, Bucks. U.K.)

Just wanted to tell you how I cured a really bad burn with your Aloe Vera. Really thought it was a hospital case & very painful. Remembering the facts in your booklet, I was delighted that the pain went almost immediately and the burn has healed quickly and without a scar. I do feel everyone should know about this, it really is miraculous.
Sincerely,
Julia L.

CANCER:

Dear Sir,
In recent months I have been receiving treatment for Breast Cancer. This has involved Radiotherapy & Chemotherapy Therapy.

I fortunately crossed paths with one of your managers, she recommended your products, in particular the Aloe Vera Nectar. I have taken this over the last 5 weeks with amazing results. The hospital had warned me that the treatment would make me feel very low. This normally happens around the 4 week mark. I am now in week 6 & am BUZZING. A new lease of life. The doctor is amazed at the lack of burning of my skin. I can only put this down to the Aloe Vera Nectar.

I have recommended to other patients who are just about to start Radiotherapy. We hope with some successful results.

yours sincerely.

Mrs. Sandra J. W. (Surrey, U.K.) 14th May,1994.

DIABETES:

Dear John& Joanne,

Thankyou for introducing me to Forever Living Products, they have had an amazing effect on my life.

Firstly, as you know I have diabetes; and since drinking the "gel" each day there have been some marked improvements in my well-being over the last three months. Probably the most profound affect is that I have had to cut my insulin intake by half, which has allowed me to reduce my weight steadily and balance my glucose levels at a more acceptable level.

Back in 1974 I broke my back in an accident which resulted in some permanent nerve damage. The consequences were I suffered a condition known as "foot drop" in the right foot and loss of feeling in the right thigh and calf. I was fitted with a caliper below the knee to support my leg and foot. Over the years my leg became weaker and I suffered a venal collapse in the lower right leg which caused me excruciating pain when walking even short distances - my consultant physician told me there was nothing that could be done, except an operation to kill the nerve supply to the area. He also added that he didn't want to take this drastic measure as I was a diabetic.

Surprise, surprise! The "gel" with its natural anti-inflammatory properties has allowed me to discard my caliper and the pain has completely gone and I can now walk the golf course with no ill effect.

Once again thankyou both very much and I have no hesitation in recommending the "Forever Living" product range to others.

Yours sincerely,
Ian W. (Northampton, U.K.) 20th July, 1994.

DERMATITIS:

I am writing to let you know how I am getting on with a dermatitis which causes the skin on my forehead and cheeks to become highly inflamed, followed by shedding of the skin.

This as you can understand has caused personal embarrassment and after using almost every cream available, thought my only real option was to use a Hydrocortisone Cream, which I was strongly against. After using the Aloe Jojoba Shampoo, it relieved my itching scalp after the first wash, and with continued regular use my scalp is now clear.

Obviously pleased with the results I decided to try both the Aloe Propolis Cream and the Aloe Gelly, on my face. The Propolis cream is extremely effective when my skin threatens to flare up. Its rich and creamy consistency does not irritate and it is very soothing.

The Aloe Gelee (Author : something that you use in the bath/shower) is wonderful, I use it both morning and evening and it has kept my skin clear and healthy for several weeks. One of my work colleagues commented on how well my skin looked lately - coming from him that was a real compliment!

These products, together with the Aloe soap are now part of my personal grooming kit, and I would have no hesitation in recommending the products.

Yours sincerely,

Les W. (Staffordshire, U.K.)

ECZEMA:

I have found the ointment to be a most excellent product. It has cleared up my husband's eczema, which had not responded to other conventional treatment, also healing for burns or cuts or abrasions is just amazing as it heals without leaving any marks. I have recommended it to other people who have also agreed with me as to its usefulness. I have been using this product myself for over five years.
Leeds,(U.K.)

Dear John,
I have suffered from eczema for 7 years and it has driven me mad at times. I have tried all the creams on the market and got fed up of booking appointments with doctors when it has not helped at all.

Since I have been using the Propolis cream my eczema has completely vanished. I am so pleased and at last I can sleep all night.
Thankyou very much for your help. I am most grateful, yours faithfully,

Mrs. Margaret L. (Worcester, U.K.)

PSORIASIS:

My son George, is 12 now. When he was four years old he began to get some dry scaly patches of skin on his body which was diagnosed as Psoriasis.
He was prescribed many and varied treatments from our G.P. all to no avail. The condition continued to worsen until by the time he was nine his body was 60% covered in Psoriasis, and he was travelling to Addenbrookes Hospital in Cambridge to be seen by their own dermatologists.
He was losing hair by this time and suffering from all associated trauma involved with that. His hands were the most badly effected, however, and he became unable to keep up with any written work at school. George's hands were white and scaly, and his fingers and thumbs were curled inwards. He was unable to straighten them at all. From time to time throughout the day and night they would crack and bleed and he would become distressed quite often.
George was incredibly lucky to have a lap-top computer donated to him by his school so that he could get on with some written work, and it worked wonders for him.
Three months ago I heard about the properties of Aloe Vera. George, by this time totally skeptical, reluctantly agreed to try it. He drank 2ozs of juice every morning and started applying Aloe Propolis Creme four times a day.

After eight weeks he had new hands. He now proudly shows off long straight fingers with new healed skin on them. He can join in with all the racquet and bat sports that he wasn't able to play before, and enjoys all art and craft activities which were previously out of the question.

It took Aloe Vera only eight weeks to treat a condition George had suffered with for eight years.

His only worry is that his school may re-claim is laptop now that he can write again!

Elizabeth W. (Lidlington, Berks, U.K.)

Dear Mr. Griffin,

I have suffered psoriasis for 20 years, tried all types of medication, been in and out of hospital several times with the condition. I was so pleased to try Forever Living Products the cream was very soothing and helped to heal my skin. At the moment I am clear from psoriasis. I am also taking Methatricate & Folic Acid.

Thankyou for your help and trust.

Eight weeks ago I couldn't even hold a pen to write this short letter.

J.M.M. (U.K.)

VETERINARY:-

Dear Jayne and John,

Having recently joined the F.L.P. team, I became very interested in the treatment of animals with Aloe Vera.

One of the most exciting results was in a treatment of an 8 month-old foal with a condition called epephysitis, an inflammation of the growth plate, causing the fetlock joint to separate and not fuse together, with resulting discomfort and bad action. Instead of using the prescribed drug, I rubbed Heat Lotion into the joint about four times each day and added 4 fluid ounces of Aloe Vera Gel to the drinking water. The vet revisited after 5 weeks and gave the foal a clean bill of health and since the foal is bred for jumping, it now has every chance of becoming a future "International".

I also treated a dog with a badly torn pad, to the base of the nail (which fell out), becoming "nasty" and pussed. I thoroughly cleaned the pad with Activator and then packed it with Aloe Vera Gelly (which gave her instant relief) and then bandaged it. This was repeated four times daily for two days, then with just the Gelly. The bandage was left off after 5 further days of treatment but I again continued with the Gelly (most of which she licked off) and the healing carried on. One week later she walked properly - no Vet or large bill!!

We also have an arthritic old terrier that now has life a lot easier, thanks to Aloe Vera Gel in her dinner every night, and the Aloe Veterinary Formula has been a great success for cuts and skin irritations.

Yours sincerely,
Amanda McG.(Bucks, U.K.)

"COMBINATION" HEALING AND RECOVERY:-

Dear Mr.St.Clair-Ford,
You asked me about any research results we may have on the Aloe Juice. Well up to date I have found it excellent in reducing pain and swelling in arthritis patients when accompanied with our herbal arthritis formula. I use it as part of our Natural Health programme for Cancer

patients, mainly to supply essential nutrients. It is amazing with viral infections, thrush etc.
I recently had personal experience of using the juice because on January 3rd '89 I had a bad fall and fractured my right hip. I had to have a hip replacement operation. I took the Aloe Juice to the hospital (Private hospital so there was no opposition) and took 20mls. morning and evening. After 4 days I was off pain killing injections and there was very little swelling of the hip and leg. The nursing staff were interested and impressed. I hope this is helpful. If you require further information do not hesitate to contact me.
Sincerely,
Nicola   K.B.Ed.(Hons)   M.H.   M.I.I.R.   N.F.S.H.
Medical Herbalist/Reflexologist. 17th February, 1989.
(Cheshire, U.K.)

Also from N.K. (Cheshire, U.K.)

We are finding excellent results with Aloe Vera Juice in the following conditions: Anti inflammatory condition, Arthritis, Sciatica, Skin disorders, Post surgical recovery, Hip replacements, knee replacements, local application to deep leg ulcers, severe mouth ulcers, tonic for general debility.

Dear Mr. Greene,

I am writing to you to tell you of my successes with the products supplied to me by your company. I first learned of the Aloe Vera Gel from my sister-in-law in Ireland, who recommended it to my wife Katherine, for the condition she was suffering from "eczema".

Upon our return to this country I purchased your "Combi-pack" of product for my wife to try. She used the gel and the propolis creme and over a period of time she realised that her condition was healing ie.4-5 weeks. She was urging me to try the aloe gel for a recurring ulcer I had for which I used Zantac prescribed by my doctor. I knew zantac wasn't good for my overall health but when one is in bad pain, one will try anything.

I found myself reaching for the Aloe Vera Gel in the early hours of the morning, doubled up with pain, and with my present supply of zantac depleted. Upon drinking the Aloe Vera I found the pain immediately went. I had experienced this with zantac but not with something as natural as a plant. I was impressed.

I took two ounces per day and also when ever I got the pain. Over the next three weeks my ulcer was gone. I know this because I went without food for twenty four hours. For those people who suffer with ulcers they know that you cannot go twenty four hours without food and not suffer great pain and discomfort.

I strongly recommend these products to any person finding themselves with this or any other ailment. If you have any questions please do not hesitate to call me.

Yours thankfully,

Brendan S. 24:05:93
(Middlesex, U.K.)

Dear Sir,

My problem started off with a persistent dry cough. My G.P. recommended me to a specialist at the local hospital who then proceeded to carry out many tests. E.N.&T. first to check throat etc., followed by the medical tests. X-ray on chest, scan, breathing test to check lungs, acidity in the gullet, twice in the theatre under anaesthetic to survey the stomach, all proved not a problem. A blood test proved satisfactory. This is now into the fourth year seeing quite a number of different doctors at the same hospital. I am very careful with what I eat, fried foods are out, hot spicy foods are out, drinks, alcohol "spirits" cannot touch. Small glass of white or red wine will be alright.

Sometimes I am sick after eating, coughing brings it on. After 4 years of this you can see no improvement in my condition, each hospital visit a different doctor would prescribe up to three lots of tablets to take before and after meals, last thing at night etc. All or most of which had some reaction to my body. Feeling high, itching skin, swollen up legs, really irritable and never getting a full nights sleep. I am still under the hospital going in again to see the doctor early January 1993.

We got to hear of Aloe Vera through my family who recommended we try it......I decided to buy the 1 litre container of Gel. Taking it by the wine glass last thing at night and first thing in the morning. The first thing that I noticed was that I slept right through the night, not waking up to cough at all and felt much better in myself throughout the day. I've not got any build up of thick yellow saliva lying in the back of my throat which eventually would make me sick.

I can only say it is a great improvement on my general state of health but if I stop taking the gel for a day or so my persistent cough comes back. Its not a complete cure but any product that will control the acid in my lower stomach and obviously is much better than taking tablets that have no effect at all. I will continue to take the gel until I have an appointment in the hospital early January and inform them of what I have been taking myself.

yours,

M.I.F. (Hampshire, U.K.) 14th December 1992.

Dear Dustin,

I am writing to let you know the results of giving my Father the Aloe Gel drink!

Do you remember I asked you if I could give my Father the drink safely as he had been suffering so much over the last 6 months with digestive problems which were also linked to the pancreas and the colon? He had been diagnosed as having gall stones too.

Last year he died twice and my Mother had to bring him back to life, so I was really anxious about giving him something that might worsen the condition. I knew he needed something and was feeling desperate to find the right thing. You advised me to try the product and I had read that were no contra-indications. You looked me straight in the eyes and said "Hand on heart, it will do him no harm." I said "O.K. I'll try it and see how he gets on." "You bet." was your reply. I went away and gave Dad the drink when I got home.

Since then Dad has had a colonectomy, which is the removal of part or all of the colon. They also discovered a large gallstone which they also removed. They performed tests on a lump they found in the colon. A few days later they told us it was cancer but they feel that they have removed all the cancer now, hopefully!

The Gel however has continued to be taken by Dad whilst in hospital and the nurses and doctors cannot understand why he is recovering so quickly. I know! He said that every time the Gel goes down, he feels instant relief from any pain or discomfort he is feeling. The wounds are healing well too!

I love my Father very much and I feel that the Forever Living Products have helped him greatly, I would just like to say thankyou for trusting in the products so much to encourage me to try the products to help my Father through a very difficult time in his life.

I personally feel, at last, that Dad has a fighting chance to continue the rest of his life in less pain than he has been experiencing lately.

May anybody who is in need of some product to help their discomfort, read this and get some hope for their conditions.

Best wishes,
Kay A. (Bucks, U.K.)

Following a road accident over 3 years ago, I badly broke the two main bones in my forearm. During the first operation I had plates and pins inserted. Eight weeks after the accident one of the bones had healed, but I had to have 3 operations on the other bone together with bone grafts which were very painful. I had my third operation in February and was in plaster for seven months because the bone would not heal again. I then had another bone graft in September. During October I heard of Lily. During my first visit she suggested I take Aloe Vera Gel which I have taken every day. Six weeks later I had my plaster removed. My doctor could not believe it. I have Lily and Aloe Vera Gel to thank.
Mr. Baily. Dec. 1993.

Dear Liz,

I initially bought Aloe Vera gelly to treat mouth ulcers but I've since found it successful in treating all sorts of ailments - toothache, cuts, spots, heat rash, even puffy eyes after a late night. It's brilliant at tightening those lines and wrinkles!

I could not be without it now. Aloe Vera Gelly really is a "bathroom" essential - I'd strongly recommend it.

Chrissie J. (Portsmouth, U.K.)

CHAPTER 7
USING ALOE VERA

I said in the introduction of this book that the problem I had with writing it was that of (in)credibility. By now, having read the varied list of testimonies, you might be thinking that what you have been reading is far fetched, that it is not possible for one product to have such an effect on so many different conditions, illnesses and ailments. If you are one of these people then there are two points to note. Point one is that you are definitely not alone in thinking this way. When my wife was talking to me about Aloe Vera and the different areas that it is effective in, it started to irritate me. My attitude was that if she wanted to believe, unconditionally that this plant could do all this, then more fool her. When I told my father that I was going to write a book about Aloe Vera, having never heard of it himself he also became irritated. He wanted to know how I could justify making all these claims? All I can do is to state that what you have read is true. I have either met the people who wrote these letters or I have met and discussed them with the people to whom they were sent. Either way, I know them to be true.

So that's the first point. Point two is that, if you are having trouble believing the testimonials then you may well "flip out" when you see what is in store for you now!

During the process of gathering these testimonials, it was clear that the amount of ailments was seemingly endless. It wasn't until I compiled a list of all the conditions that I have either witnessed or heard that Aloe Vera has had regular success with that I found myself looking at a list that defies belief.

i) **Illnesses/conditions/ailments that Aloe Vera has regularly benefited:** *Please note, this does not mean cure, it means that relief has been experienced to varying degrees.* Please note, I must repeat that if you are suffering from any ailment or condition, or you are on medication of any kind, consult your doctor.

A: Acne, aching joints & muscles, asthma, athletes foot, abscesses, arthritis, allergy rashes, age spots, acid indigestion, asthma.

B: Brown skin spots, burns, boils, blood pressure, bruising, bad breath, bleeding, bowel problems/conditions, blisters, bronchitis.

C: Cancer treatment, (ie. helps ease the radiation effects), cuts & wounds, colon cleansing, constipation, calcium, Crohn's disease, chapping, cataracts, cradle cap, cystitis, candida, circulation, colitis, colic.

D: Digestive problems, diarrhoea, dermatitis, dandruff, diabetes, detoxification, duodenal ulcer, diaper (nappy) rash, denture sores, depression.

E: Eye and ear problems, (inflammation, infection), eczema, energy loss.

G: Gum disease, bleeding gums.

H: Hair & scalp, heat rash, haemorrhoids, headache, herpes.

I: Infection, inflammation, itching, Irritable bowel syndrome, indigestion, insomnia, influenza, insect bites.

J: Jaundice.

K: Kidney ailments.

L: Liver ailments, laryngitis.

M: Moisturises, M.E., mouth ulcers, muscle cramps.

N: Nasal congestion, nutrition, nappy (diaper) rash, cracked nipples, nausea.

O: Recovery from operations, oral disorders.

P: Psoriasis, prickly heat, pimple, peptic ulcer, pain relief.

R: Radiation burns, razor burn, rheumatism, rashes.

S: Scar removal, scalp problems, sinusitis, sore throat, scalding, stomach disorders, sciatica, strains, sprains, skin problems, stress, shingles, stings, styes, sunburn, sores of all kinds.

T: Tonsillitis, thrush, teething, tennis elbow.

U: Ulcers, (all kinds.)

V: Varicose veins, veterinary treatments, venereal sores.

W: Warts, wind chapping.

So there's the list! Eleven months ago I found this kind of information offensive to the point of irresponsibility. It wasn't right, I thought, for people to be given false hope with so many different conditions. Where was the proof that this "magical" plant could bring relief to so many conditions? Having been researching for this book, having used Aloe Vera on myself and family and felt the relief that it has given and the sense of well-being, having spoken to people from all walks of life and with totally differing attitudes who have experienced the same, I find myself almost feeling ashamed of having had those feelings. This may sound a little strong, even a little melodramatic. How can I seem to be emotional when talking about a plant? For me it is more than just the plant itself, it offers a possibility of relief and freedom from suffering, in some cases where all else has failed and after years of affliction. It offers Quality of Life to almost everyone. Just take another look at the list and tell me that you don't know anyone who is suffering from at least one of these conditions. I don't believe that you can. It might even be you. Then imagine all those people with all those conditions relieved of their suffering, with no side effects, short or long term, no toxins and no addiction. That to me is what this is about.

ii) How Aloe Vera is used.

With so many conditions that Aloe Vera appears helpful for, it seems appropriate to find out in what form it comes and how it is taken.

First of all though, there are a few "pointers" to look out for. Aloe Vera can come in powder form, or dehydrated and then re-hydrated. My personal reaction to this as with any natural produce is that "fresh is best". This is born out in an account that I read about where a doctor was using fresh Aloe on a patient and, during the course of the treatment, ran out. As he had no further fresh supplies, he used powdered Aloe Vera which, although it worked, had a significantly reduced level of healing rate. Although I accept that there are many variants in a one off example I stress that this is very much a personal stance.

The second point to look out for is the percentage of Aloe Vera in the product. There is an increasing amount of produce, particularly in the cosmetic range, that includes Aloe Vera in its ingredients. The difference between them and the companies that specialise in Aloe Vera produce is that the cosmetic's may have, at best a few percent Aloe Vera, at worst a fraction of one percent. This is not saying that a small percentage of Aloe Vera will not have any effect but when the specialist companies use from 70% up 100% it puts it into perspective. (By the way, would multi-national companies be using Aloe Vera and making such a big noise about it if there was nothing to it?)

The third point is to make sure that the Aloe is stabilised. This prevents the Aloe Vera from oxidising and thereby losing its potency. A good example of oxidising is when a bite is taken out of an apple and then it is left in the open. Within a few minutes it is possible to see the apple go brown as the apple oxidises. Stabilisation, however, keeps the Aloe Vera stabilised in its near fresh state. One company, Forever Living Products, has a patented stabilisation technique that allows the Aloe Vera juice to remain in its fresh state in a sealed bottle for an incredible 5 years. Once opened it will last for up to 6 months if refrigerated.

The ways of using Aloe Vera are simple enough. It can either be drunk, rubbed or sprayed on.

Aloe Vera Juice is taken internally and ranges from 97% to 99% Aloe Vera. There is no "hard and fast" rule as to how much should be taken and I must confess to finding this a little alarming at first. However, it must be remembered that this isn't a drug, it is the non-toxic juice of a plant, of which 95% is water. I draw a similarity here with taking orange juice for its vitamin C content, how much is enough?

The main factor that determines how much an individual takes is the actual reason for which it is being taken. For instance, if it is because the individual is having some intestinal spasm, then it might be necessary to take a larger initial amount in order to have an immediate and powerful effect. In my case, I took four tablespoons which sorted out the problem immediately. The following two days I took two tablespoons three times a day until there was absolutely no doubt of a recurrence.

If, on the other hand you are either taking Aloe juice to deal with a condition that has a longer duration of pain (e.g. arthritis), or flushing through an allergic reaction, or for a de-tox programme, then it is more important to maintain a steady supply of Aloe into your system. In these instances, two tablespoons in the morning an hour before breakfast and in the evening before bed would be the most recommended amount. Dr.Gregg Henderson gives patients with stomach ulcers a tablespoon an hour. It should be noted that these people are often scheduled for surgery.

Dr. Atherton recommends a maximum daily intake of 4fl.oz. (1 standard tablespoon holds 1 fl.oz.) which I think is sound advice. However, for some if it feels too much or too little they adjust the amount to what suits their feeling. As I said I was at first rather concerned about this seemingly casual approach but there was one benefit that came out of it which was that as I was monitoring myself I took far more care over what I actually needed. If this had been the doctor's tablets I would have just taken them *without a second thought*.

Many people take Aloe Vera as a tonic. I have been taking two tablespoons in the morning and two in the evening for nearly a year now. Sometimes I go through a week or so of not taking it but generally I now take it every day as a de-tox and preventative regime, simply for the reason that every day I am eating food that contains pesticides, colourings, chemicals, saturated fats etc. which needs to be combated.

Aloe Vera juice gives the body the chance to readjust, regulate and heal, affecting us at the cellular level. Some of its components have an effect on our nervous system, our ability to process food, the way we regenerate new cells, the way we heal ourselves and far more. The more constant the supply, the more it will flush out toxins that cause illness, allergic reactions and lethargy, making more energy available and a better sense of well-being, ultimately increasing the ability of the individual taking it.

Areas where it may help; almost all. This may seem a grand statement and to justify it recap on what Aloe Vera has been found to contain and the properties that go along with that. It is a natural cleanser, it penetrates tissues deeply, it relieves pain deep beneath the surface, it is antibiotic, it is anti-inflammatory, it is antipyretic, (relieving the heat associated with burns and inflammations), it is antipruritic, (relieves itching) , it is nutritional, it is an effective humectant, (it promotes the retention of water in skin tissues), it dissolves and digests dead cells and speeds up the rate of cell growth in a damaged area, thus speeding up the healing process. How can it not help almost all areas is more the point.

Aloe Vera Gelly is Aloe Vera in an easy to use gelly form, which has been prepared from the stabilised juice. The content of Aloe Vera in the gelly from the specialist suppliers of Aloe Vera produce ranges from 97% to 99.9% pure Aloe Vera.

The use of the gelly is really down to common sense. Firstly, it is for external use and can be applied to any damaged skin tissue such as cuts, burns, blisters, skin infections, itching, insect bites and stings, sunburn, acne, razor burn, allergy and other rashes, rubbed on the gum for teething troubles. It can also be applied for athletes foot and haemorrhoids.

One additional advantage is that it can be applied on a "when needed" basis. The gelly is an excellent way of illustrating the absorption power of Aloe Vera, within three to four minutes of application the gelly will have been absorbed into the skin, leaving no trace.

Aloe First Aid is a product that I find a "must" particularly with children. As with the gelly it can be used for any skin damage or irritation but the big advantage is its pump action spray. The last thing that anyone wants is to have a lotion of some kind rubbed onto a wound, burn, graze or sting! To be able to gently spray makes far more sense. This contains in the region of 90% Aloe Vera and brings instant relief.

These three that I have mentioned are the basic three products that Aloe Vera specialists tend to market. In addition there is a small range of products that are common to them which tends to be in the skin care range. The applications of these are very straight forward and do not require further explanation.

iii) Points to be aware of before using Aloe Vera:

a) Many people have an allergy to something, so it is probable that, just as some are allergic to orange juice, for example, then some may be allergic to Aloe Vera. Allergic reaction usually manifests in the form of stinging, itching, a mild rash or a combination of these with the reaction, if it is going to happen, appearing quickly. In order to check tolerance levels to Aloe Vera the best thing would be to get a pure Aloe product (like the juice or activator) and rub it on the under arm or just behind the ear. If a reaction occurs, do not use Aloe Vera.

b) When first taking the juice, some people go through a few days of feeling worse. This might be in the form of headaches, aches in general, diarrhoea, lethargy, irritability. In nearly all of these cases it is because the system is being flushed through and, in the process, all the toxins and crud that have been gathering are being disposed of. Symptoms such as athletes foot have often been present but dormant, pushed underground if you like. This way it is brought back out "into the open" where it can be dealt with permanently. In these instances an external application, such as activator and deep heat should be used to deal with the surface scenario, allowing the juice to flush the remains through the system. Working externally and internally exposes and eradicates rather than just putting a symptom "on hold." In the instance of diarrhoea, Dr. Atherton tells his patients that, if it hasn't gone in two to three days, then reduce the dose.

It is important that individuals understand this "flushing through" process and also test for allergic reaction to Aloe Vera and any possible additional ingredients. On some occasions the individual has stopped because they have been put off. Although this is understandable it is also a pity. On others they have persevered and watched a condition that had been flaring up on and off for years, disappear.

c)   If there is a reaction when using an Aloe Vera product, it is also advisable to check if there are other ingredients. There was one time when I was using an Aloe Creme that had another remarkable natural substance in it called Bee Propolis (which is a natural antibiotic). My face was suddenly stinging badly and came out in a rash. Looking at the tube I discovered that the product contained Lanolin, to which I am allergic. I immediately applied Aloe Gelly and the reaction was gone.

d)   On quite a number of occasions, people who have taken Aloe juice for a specific reason find that, without realising it, other ailments or conditions clear up. For example, a friend of mine was taking Aloe Vera juice as a general health tonic, with a more specific aim of preparing herself for an operation. After a period of around four weeks, she noticed that brown skin marks/spots on her hands had simply vanished.

e)   **Please note:** when using Aloe Vera products on cuts, grazes, basically all external damaged skin tissue, it is extremely important that the area is cleaned as much as possible. This is not only good basic medical practice but in this case because Aloe Vera penetrates all seven layers of the skin it can not only take down all its healing properties into the damaged tissue but it can also take dirt down too, which could have a harmful effect.

Once again, I repeat that those with ailments or conditions of any kind need to consult with their doctor. It is not intended for this to be a replacement for any medication.

CHAPTER 8

SELF ASSESSMENT

I mentioned in the previous chapter that there may be a number of different outcomes when using Aloe Vera. This might be the healing of an ailment or condition for which Aloe Vera has been taken, or that something else, totally unrelated, unexpectedly heals. It may simply be a feeling of well being. It often happens that changes occur and are not noticed either because the process was so subtle or because the focus was on something else. It is because of this diversity and on occasion subtleness of responses that I have included this chapter in the book. It is for those who take Aloe Vera who might want to keep their own account of what changes occur, showing any progression made. For example, there may be very small changes that on their own don't add up to much. When put together over weeks or months a full picture emerges.

What I have done is set out four questions that I believe would prompt the most relevant feedback for anyone wishing to assess their progress. For those taking part in this exercise, I would suggest making copies to cover the following routine : end of each day 1-7, because there are normally more daily changes in the first week. End of week 1-6, because six weeks is an average time for more longer term changes in conditions such as arthritis to stabilise. End of months 2 and 3, because this should be long enough for any fluctuations to have settled and a true picture to emerge. For those who maybe using Aloe Vera juice which is stored in the refrigerator, why not keep your notes on the fridge door?

In order to assess what progress is being made, it is necessary to know from where the progression starts, ie. the original symptoms, I would therefore recommend that time is taken not only to record the original symptoms but also any secondary ailments. This might not be as simple as it at first may seem because, as the word condition suggests, we become "conditioned" to certain feelings like low energy, a dull ache, dry skin or poor sleep and might not realise it. Write as much as you need, itemise it clearly and record how this symptom affects you.

When answering these questions over the next few weeks, allow yourselves a specific time to do this for two reasons: the first is that these questions require a degree of both physical and mental self - assessment. Asking how you feel does not only refer to physical symptoms, it refers to emotional ones. I believe that this is the most important element not only in healing but also our lifestyle. The second reason for setting aside a regular and specific time is that it gives a chance to just sit down and rest. In the day-to-day mayhem that is many people's lives, the one thing that most of us do not allow ourselves is time to find out how we are doing! This is particularly crazy when we are ill. So take "time out", indulge yourself!

I would expect that many people might consider this exercise a waste of time, which is fair enough. However, I regularly come across people who, when I start asking them about their general state of health, suddenly start to notice changes which, because they hadn't simply stopped to think about, they hadn't noticed. The immediate realisation that something else has cleared up without their having noticed often produces an instant increase in these people's sense of well being, as though some "block" has been removed.

PERSONAL OBSERVATION NOTES

1) Have you noticed any change in the symptoms?

2) Have there been any changes that you weren't expecting?

3) In what form(s) are you using Aloe Vera? How much and how often?

4) How have you been feeling? How do you feel now?

CHAPTER 9
IN CLOSING. . . . .

In closing there is one point in particular that I feel needs to be made. If anyone who is considering using Aloe Vera has any "niggling" doubts, then find an answer that satisfies that doubt. If it's not in this book, then talk to someone who uses Aloe Vera themselves. If I can be of any help then please write to me c/o The Wordsmith Publishing Company, 46a, West Street, Farnham, Surrey, GU9 7DX. (U.K.) It is all very well for people such as myself to praise the virtues of Aloe Vera but it is your body that you are considering applying it to. What is right for me is not necessarily right for others. However, I believe that the experiences that I and those with whom I have talked with, read and heard about are worth something, if only to show that there are always options. With the medical world turning its attention on the plant world we can be sure that there will soon be many exciting and far healthier alternatives available than that which conventional medicine has to offer today. (For instance one American organisation is screening over 10,000 plants a year.)

I stated that this book was not about persuasion or conviction. Again I reiterate this. If individuals try Aloe Vera as a result of reading this book then the only true opinion of the individual will come from that outcome, not from what has been written here. For those who do use Aloe Vera, I have a request to make. I briefly mentioned that Dr. Atherton and I are looking to compile a follow - up book on Aloe Vera in 1995. This will be more specifically documented on groups of cases. (Eg. eczema, M.E. I.B.S. psoriasis.) My request is that would anyone who uses the progress report in chapter 8 please consider sending me a copy, c/o The Wordsmith Publishing Company and mark it confidential. The more cases we study the clearer the conclusions. Thankyou in advance.

Finally, I mentioned how the main problem was writing about a bitter gelly, that is extracted from a plant that has been used by mankind for over 4,000 years and relieves an extensive list of ailments (with no side effects) and yet offers no explanation as to how it does it , whilst maintaining credibility. Up until nine days ago this was still a problem until, that is, I happened to glance at an article in my daily paper. It was about how in 1899, Bayer, the pharmaceutical company, produced a white powder which, so they claimed, reduced pain, inflammation and fever. However, no one knew how it worked but it had been used for over 2,000 years, it was refined from a bitter and sickening preparation derived from willow bark and other plants such as meadowsweet. Even now there are claims that it can protect against colorectal cancer, delay the aging process, stops H.I.V. and can prevent heart attacks.

What wild claims, I thought! Not only don't they know what made it work but it has the nasty side effect of gastro-intestinal bleeding. Who is going to take such a product seriously, let alone buy it?

The truth is all of us, over 40,000 tonnes a year of it, 100 tonnes a day, five tonnes every hour . . . . it's called aspirin!

I wish you good health.

NOTES:

NOTES:

NOTES:

NOTES:

NOTES:

NOTES: